# A
# Relaxation
# Journey

By
Kate Mullin

Illustration by Liz Mullin

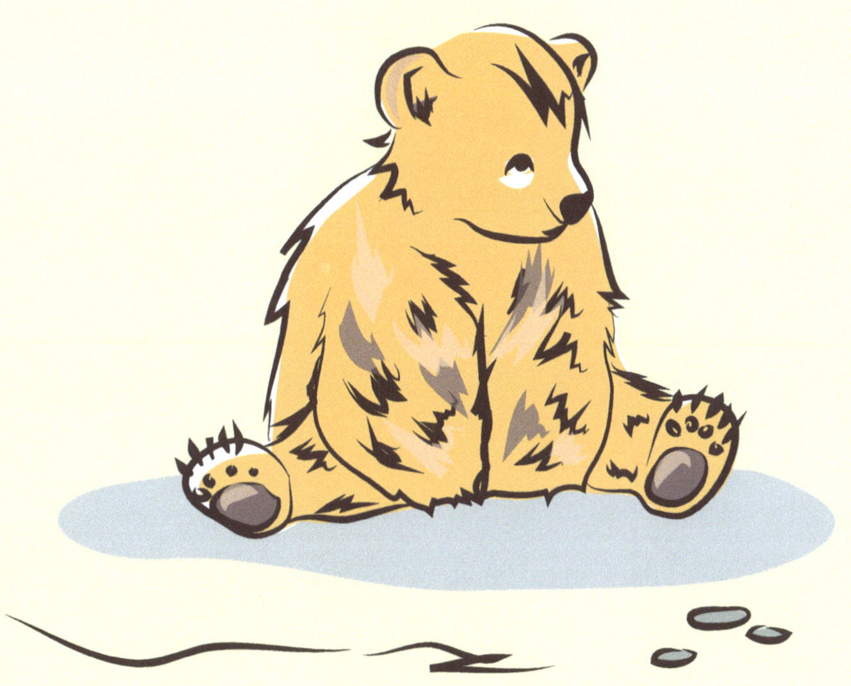

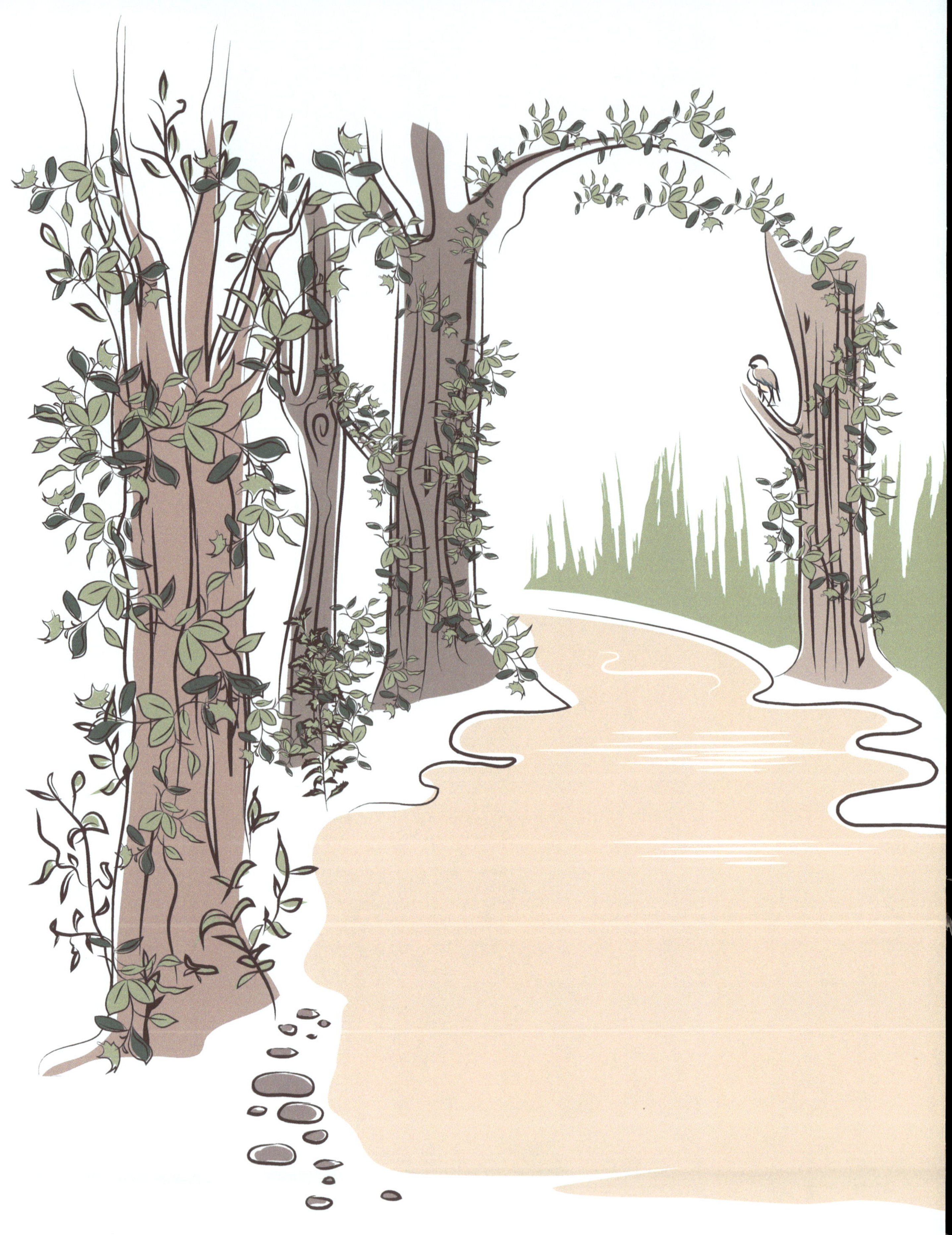

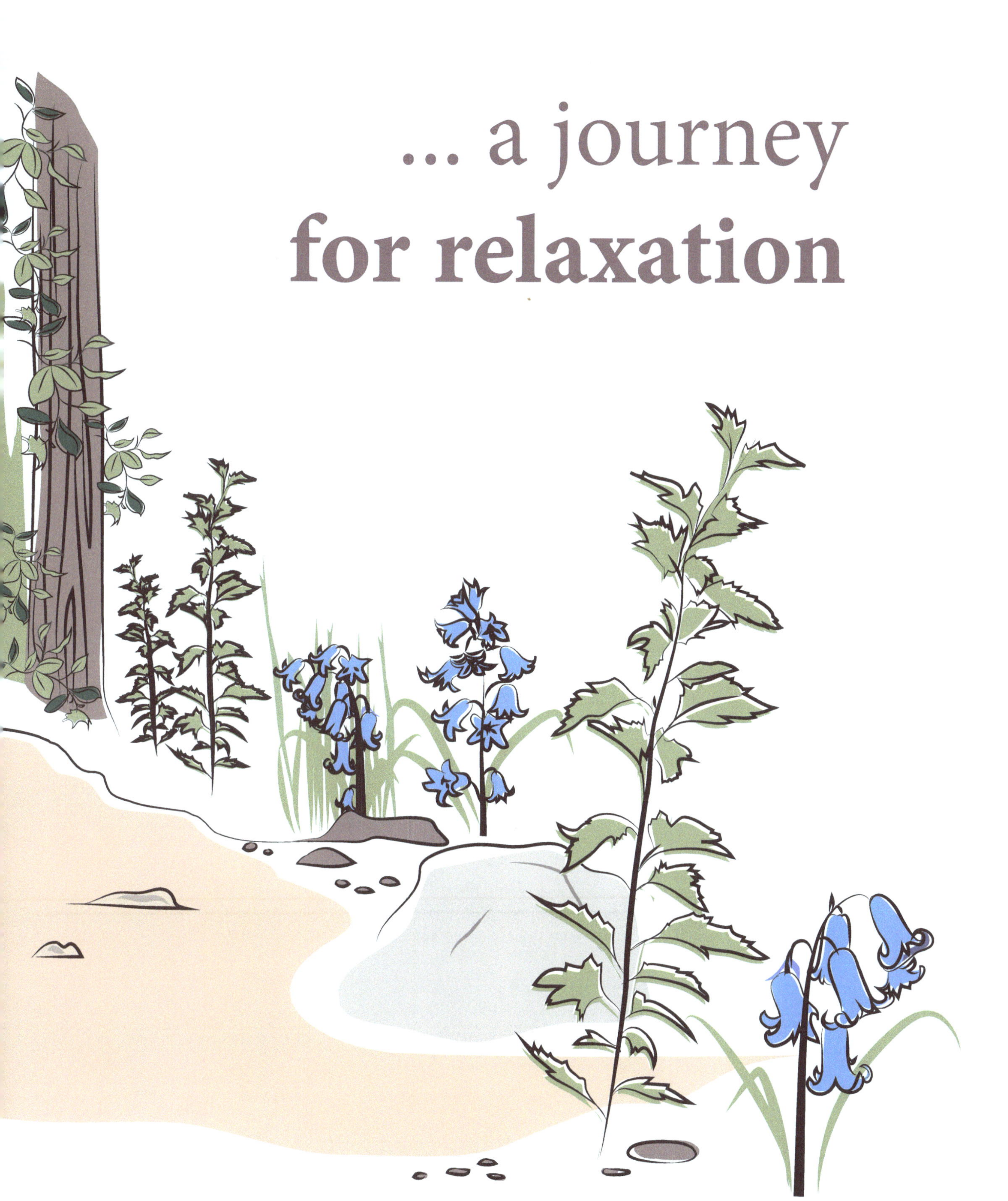
... a journey
for relaxation

Dedicated to

Bluebell Park School

First Published May 2018

# A Relaxation Journey

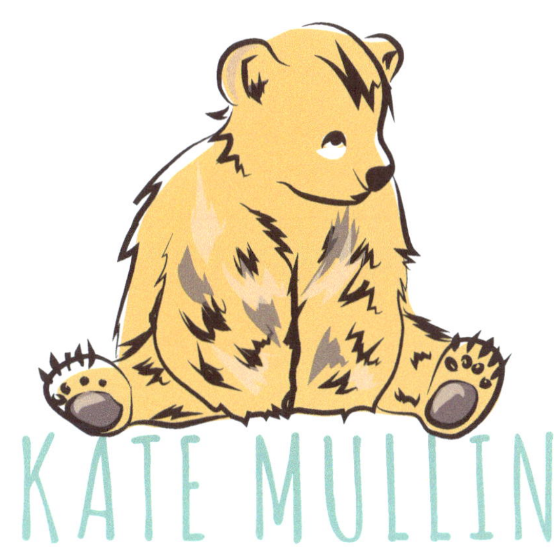

KATE MULLIN

# A Relaxation Journey

## Specially designed to help children relax.

*Information for the reader.*

This book uses relaxation techniques through a story. It is written with a special design, using language to promote relaxation. It uses a progressive muscle relaxation which helps the body to relax. The bold type is the subconscious suggestions for the mind, along with simple metaphors. Each cave represents a positive thought for the mind to program in results. It's a great way to encourage a good start to the day, or can be used to relax at the end of the day too.

*Read slowly when you see the '…' or pause for a few moments.*

*Make sure everyone is awake after the relaxation if it is during the day. Never listen when driving or doing anything with machinery.*

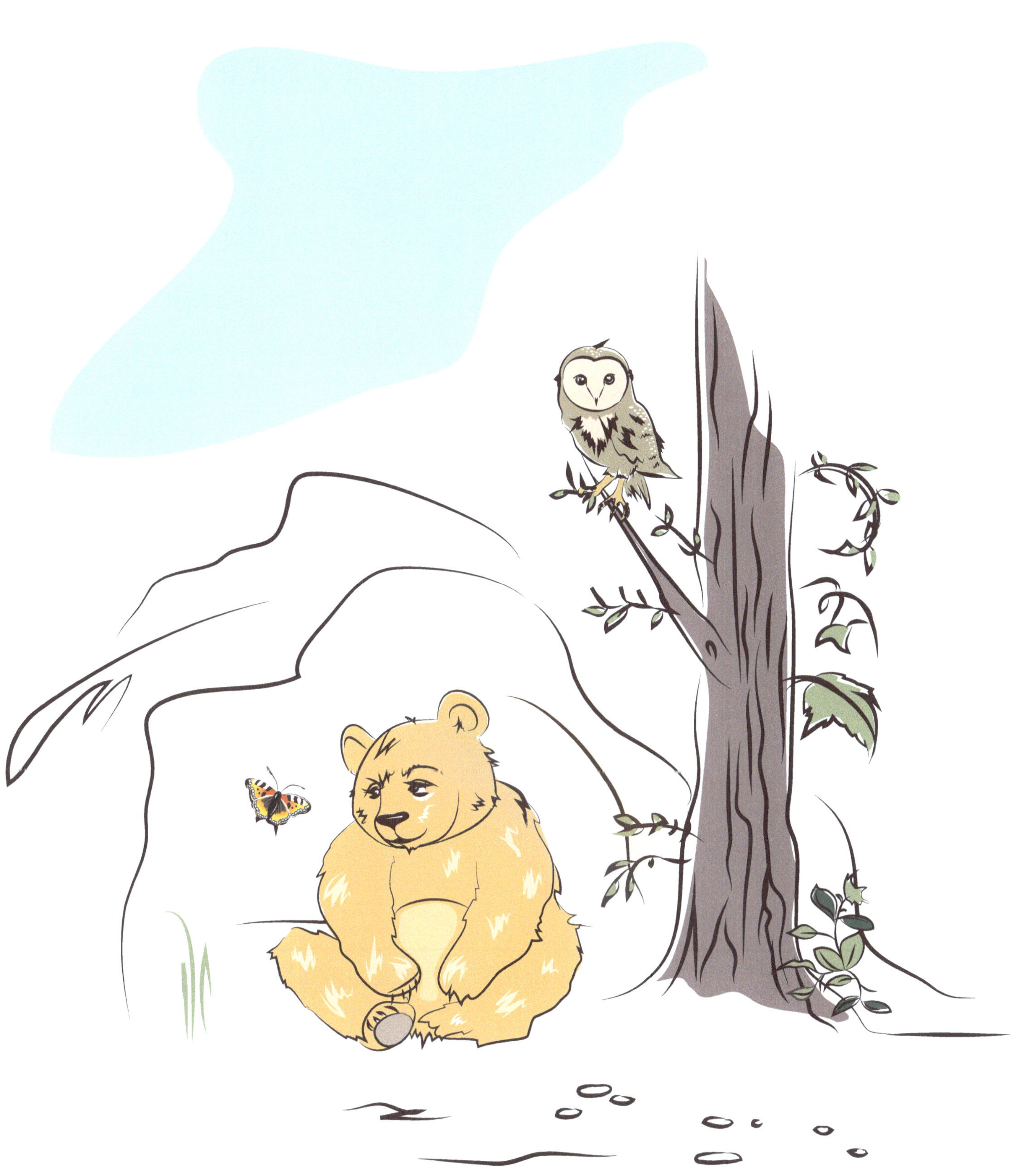

# A Relaxation Journey

I'm wondering if you're comfortable? If the answer is yes, then we can begin our relaxation story. You're going to travel to a special place with Mosey bear to the Rainbow Caves where all the secrets of relaxation **can be found.** Mosey is very special just like you. He doesn't find it **easy to relax quickly every day.** I'm wondering if you can you help him to relax? Let's begin our relaxation journey...

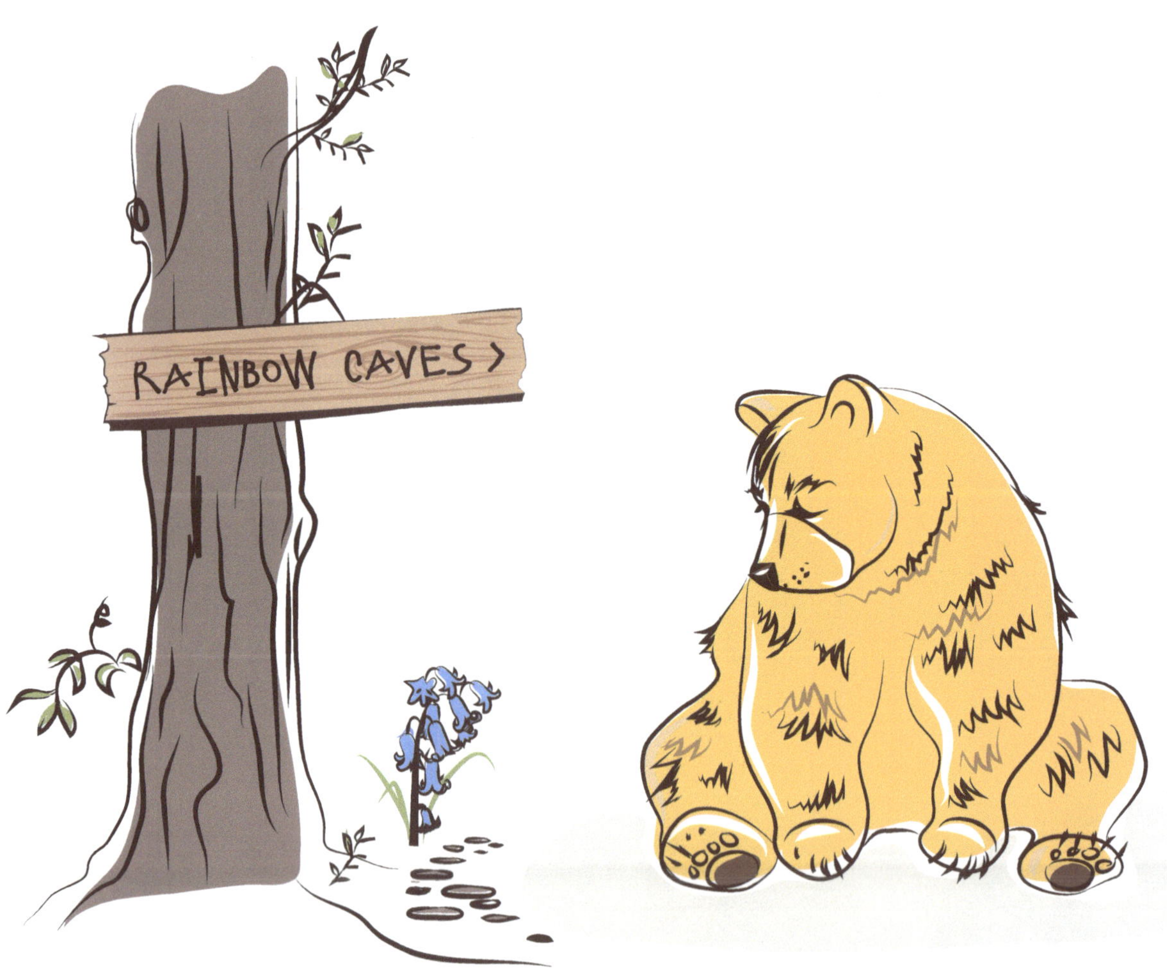

First, **listen to the sound of your heart beat.** Put your hand on your wrist and count the beats. This is a story for relaxation, so don't worry if you find that **you start to relax very easily. Listen... Can you hear** the sound of your breathing? Shhh… Some words **you will hear** while others **will float away. You will hear** the words that you need.

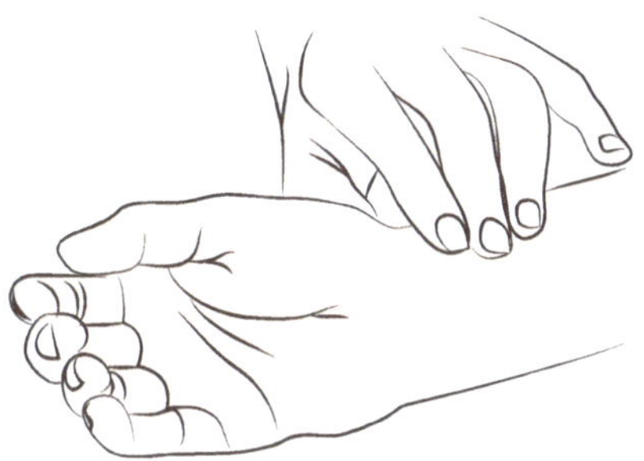

Your arms and legs might feel floaty as **you listen,** or your arms and legs might feel heavy. Can you feel happy tingles of relaxation in your body? Relax more and even deeper; feel your body let go, see how easy it feels.

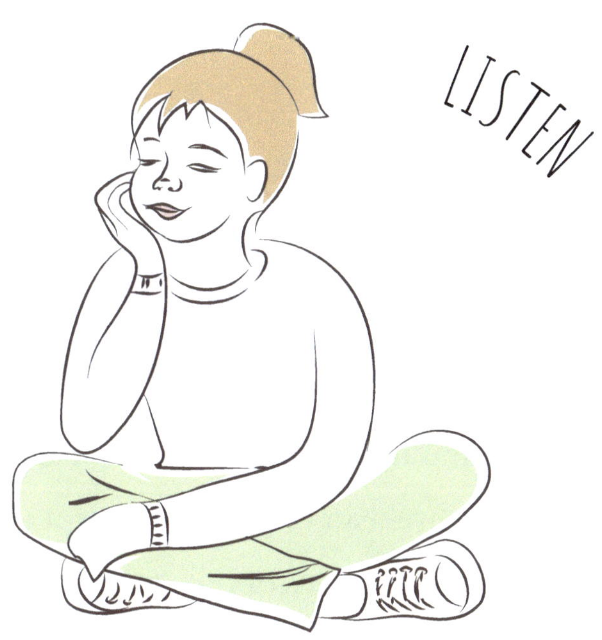

Spread the relaxation to your fingers, to your thumbs, to your wrists, to your elbows… to your arms... to your shoulders...

And now to your neck. Allow the relaxation to spread from muscle to muscle. As the relaxation spreads, you can feel your body becoming more and more happy, relaxing tingles all around; your arms and legs float and help you to relax.

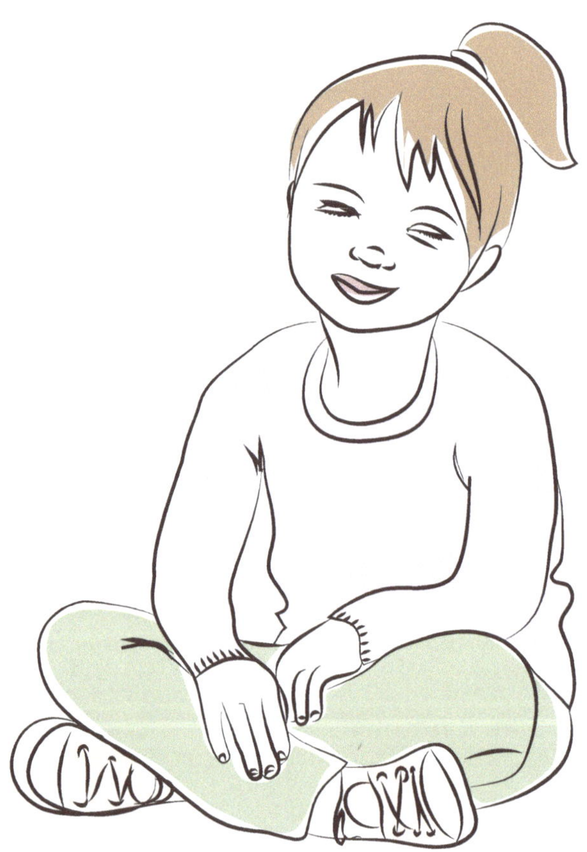

Relax your face; your mouth can be a little bit apart, your jaw is loose and relaxed. Feel your forehead relaxing, wiggle it around to check. Smile and feel those happy tingles of relaxation.

Now relax your tummy, relax your spine, relax your chest.
Relax your hips and as you float deeper, relaxing every part of you;
relax your knees... relax your ankles... and every toe, including the
middle toe of your right foot. And as your body relaxes, your mind
will also relax now too. Switch off thoughts. Don't worry if they still
happen, just let them wander far away.

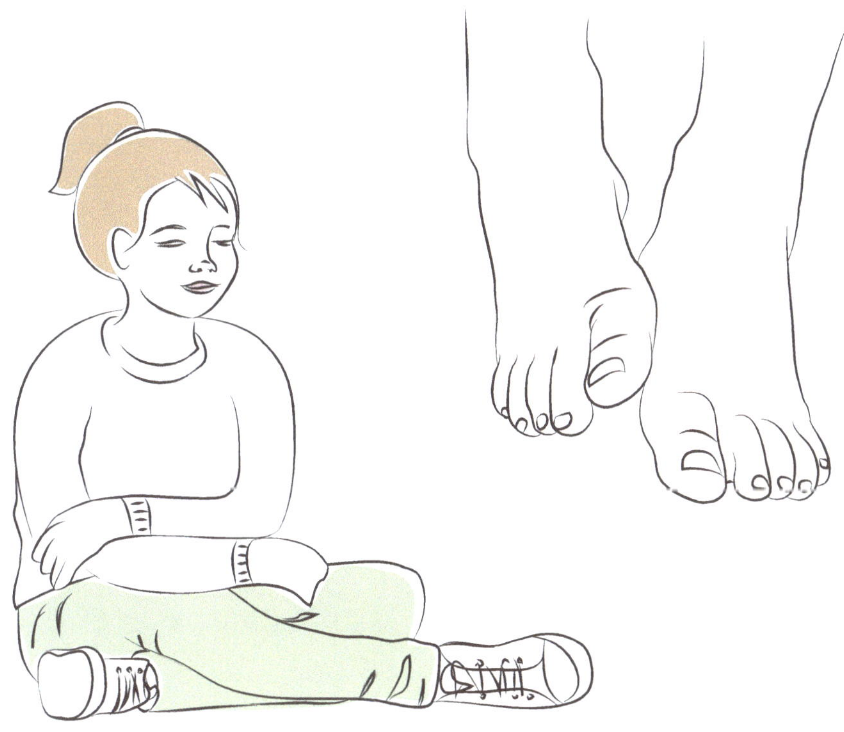

As you **listen, you feel new relaxing sensations arrive** all the time.
Mosey bear is so happy to **know you are relaxing too**. You can
**discover the answers to relaxing together** in the Rainbow Caves with
Mosey bear.

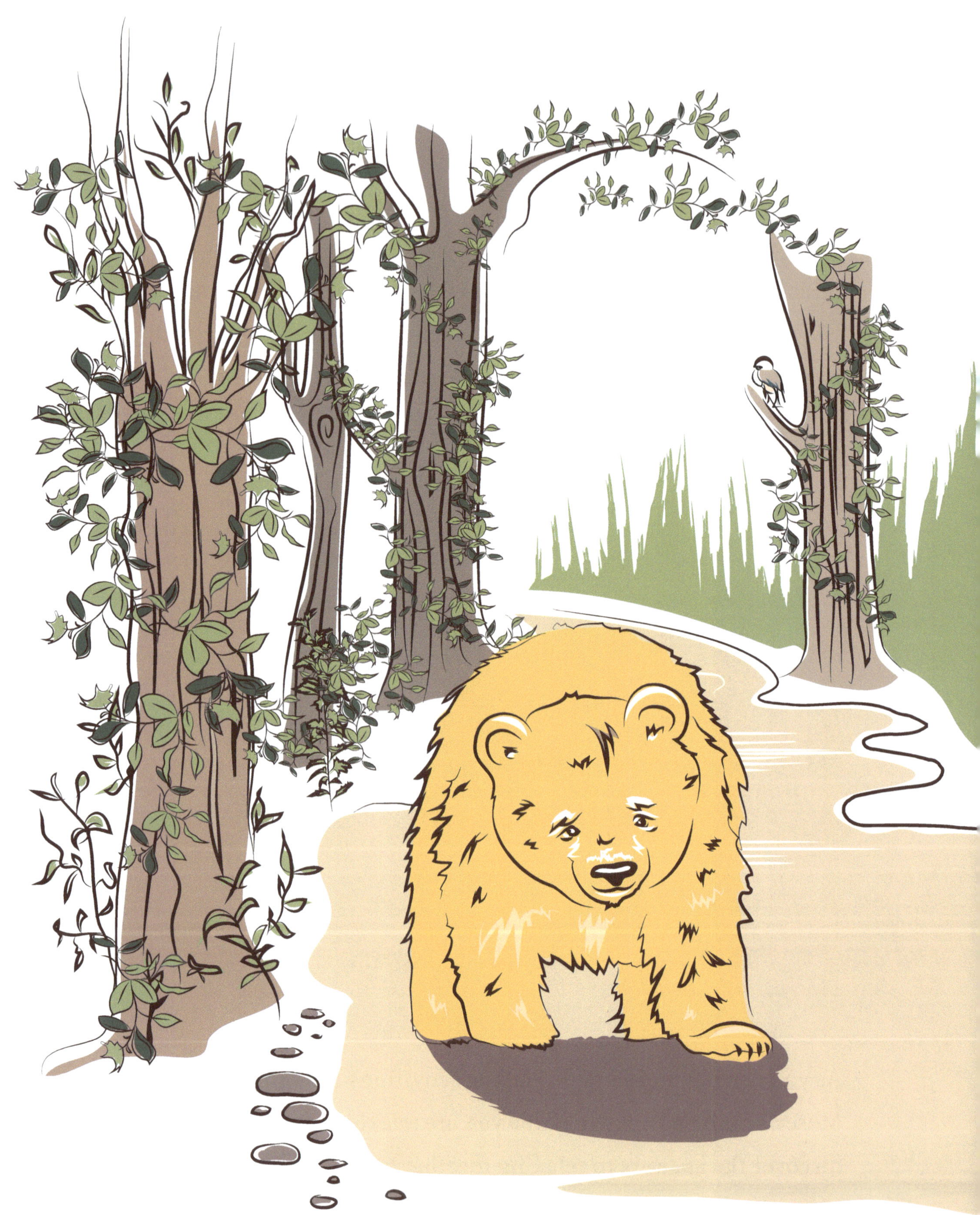

Let's wander along...

All you have to do is **relax**, like a leaf falling from a tree.

See it drift down.

"**Let's wander** to the Rainbow Caves!" says Mosey bear.


**Close your eyes** whenever you want to.

Use your imagination (a picture in the mind)

to see a lovely forest in front of you.

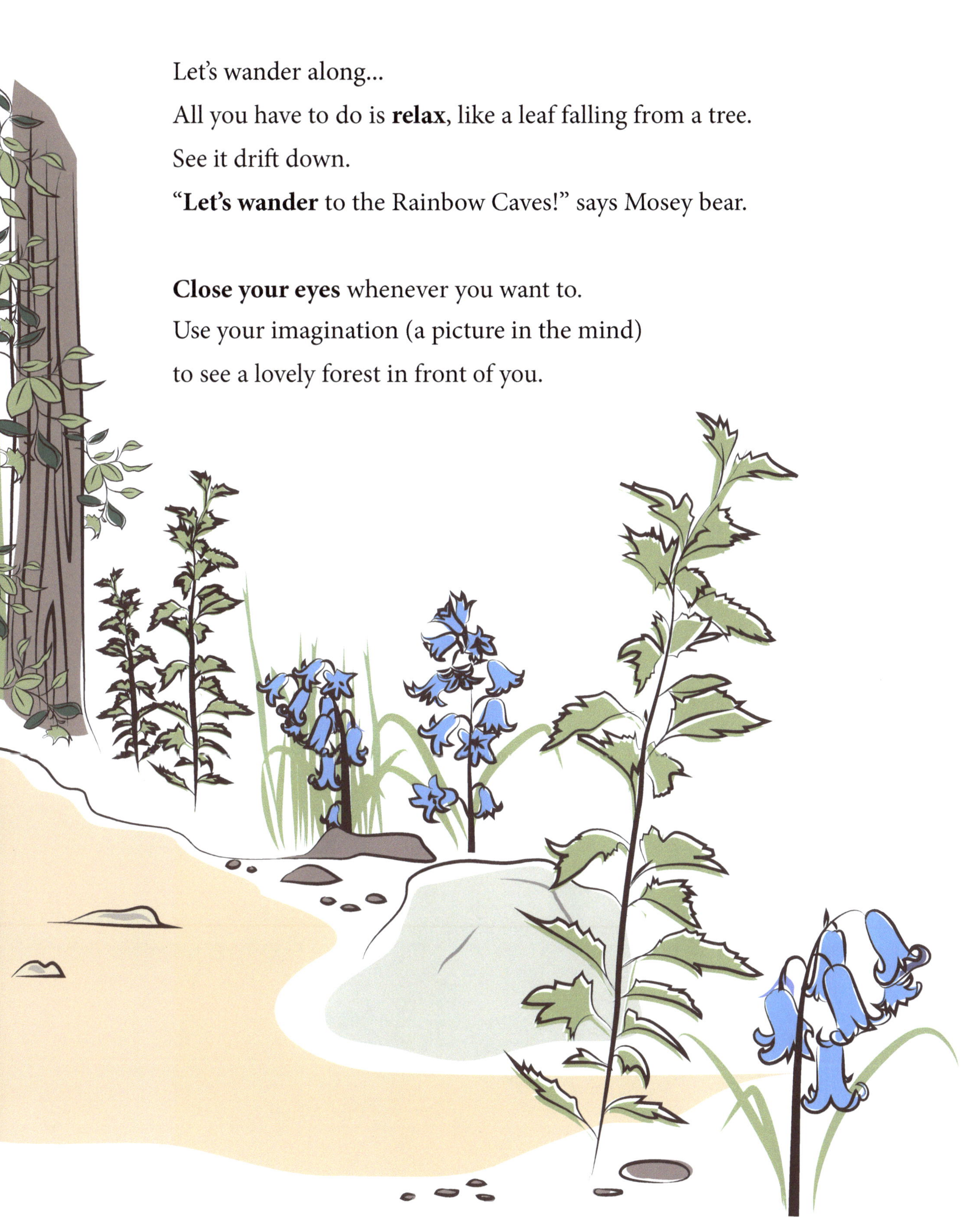

This is the most beautiful forest you can imagine. Mosey bear walks ahead and you follow. You can hear birds singing and leaves rustling as the sun shines on your face. You walk along and follow the path. You notice trees with leaves as big as parachutes and berry fruits as large as footballs. You notice trees and woodland sounds; like birds singing and woodland creatures playing. You feel alive and smell the fresh air. Butterflies surround you as you wander further. You have tingles of happiness in this forest, as every step you take fills you with wonder. You see a sign ahead for the Rainbow Caves.

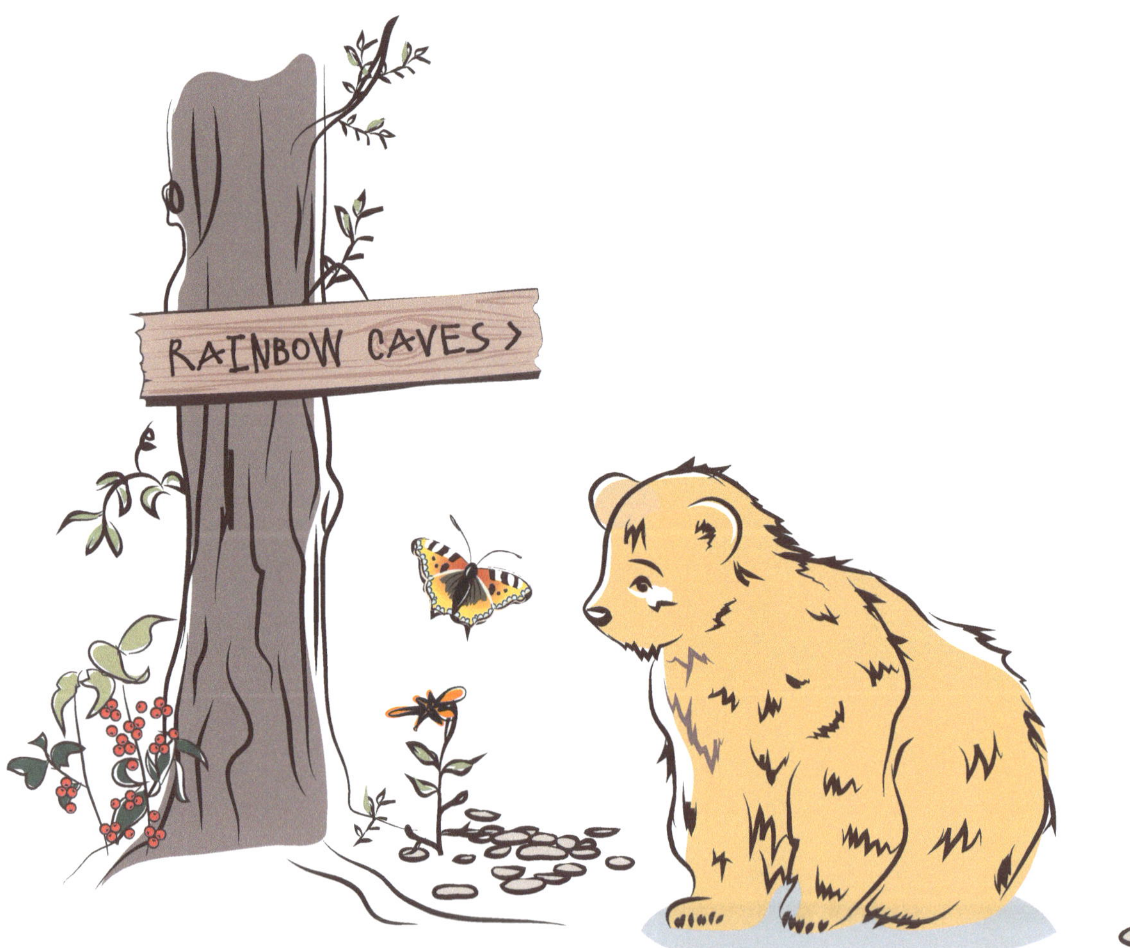

Birds fly high above you to see you on your way. Mosey bear waves to you to **keep going**. Tiny dragon flies with lights on their tails guide you. Then up ahead as the trees and forest ends, you see the first Rainbow Cave.

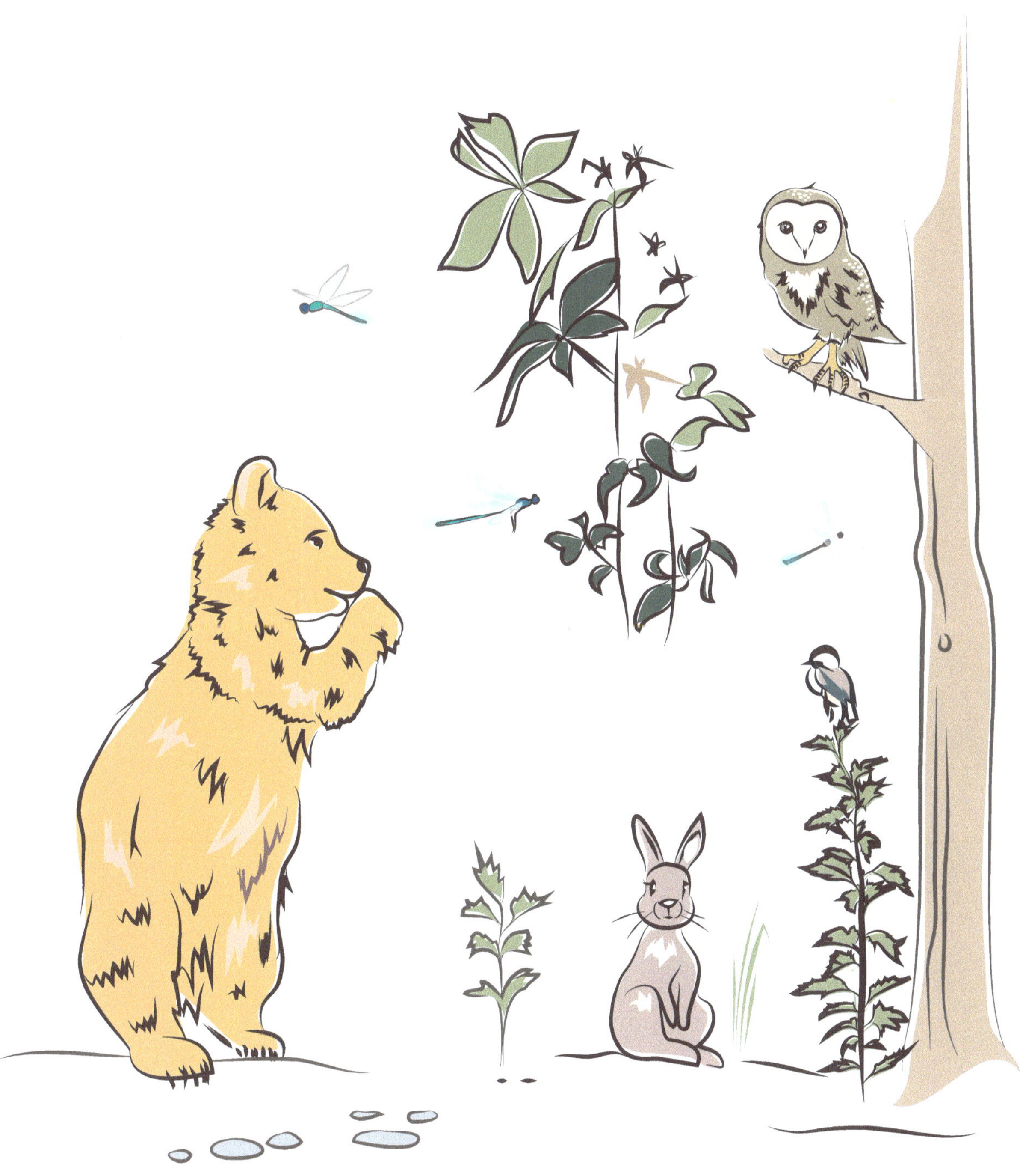

The first cave is the red cave.

Everything in here is a relaxing red colour.

It has a warm red glow.

It feels so cosy.


The Rainbow Caves will **help you along** the way.

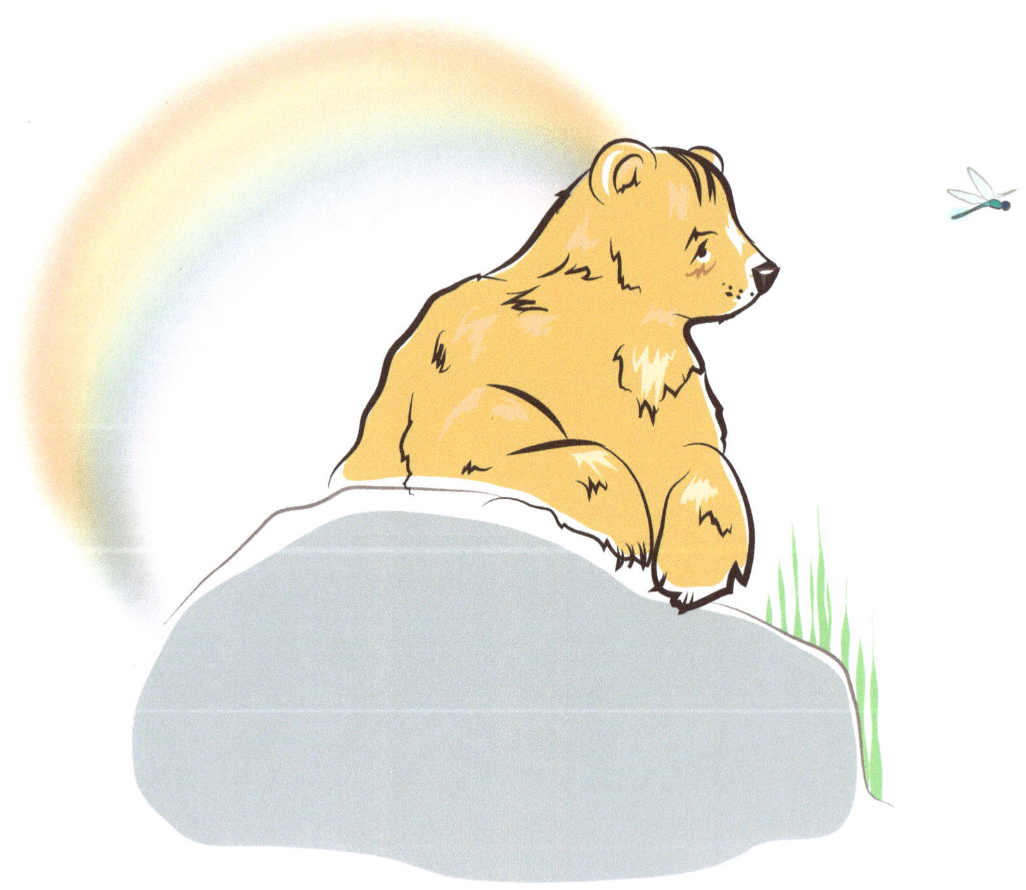

In the red cave you follow Mosey. Relax and look around. You see everything is a warm red and makes you feel toasty and safe.

**You feel safe and confident.**

Take anything you need.

Take the confidence you feel in here with you at all times.

You have the confidence to **relax.**

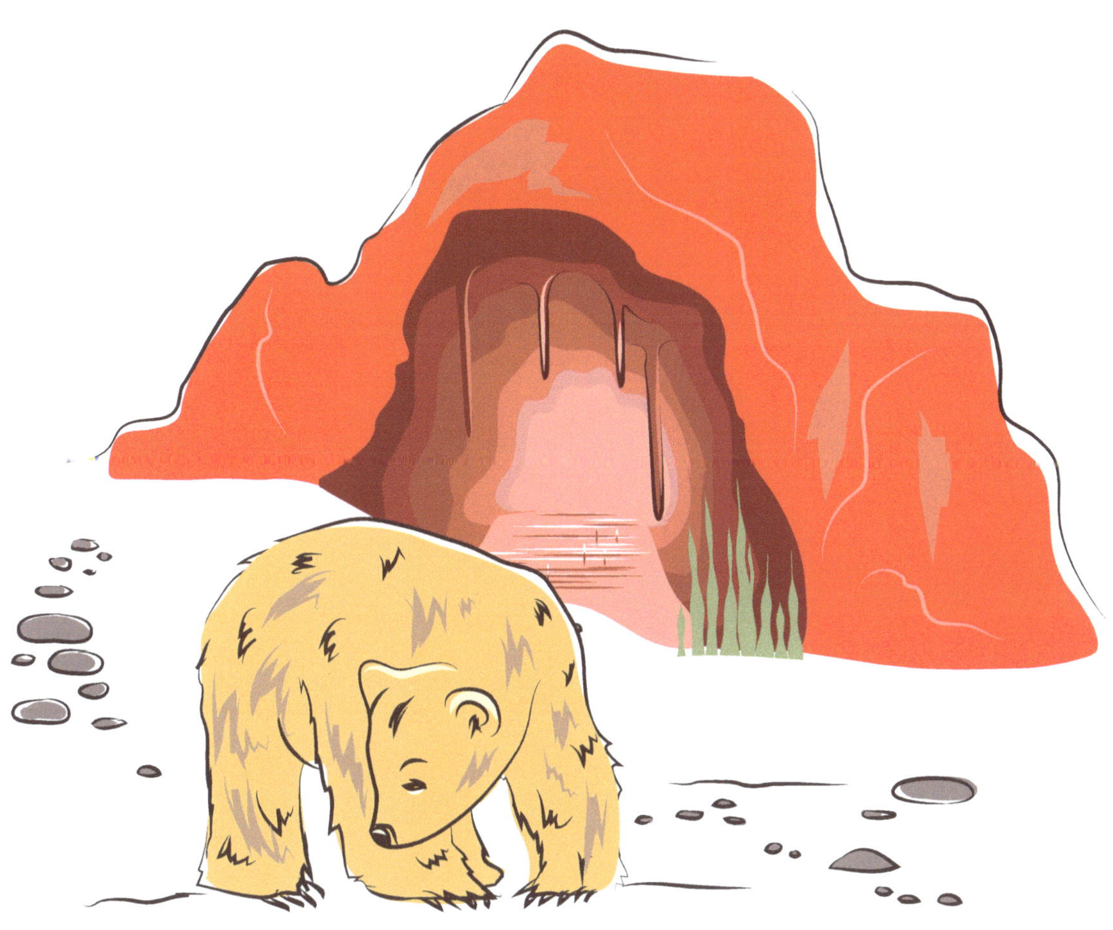

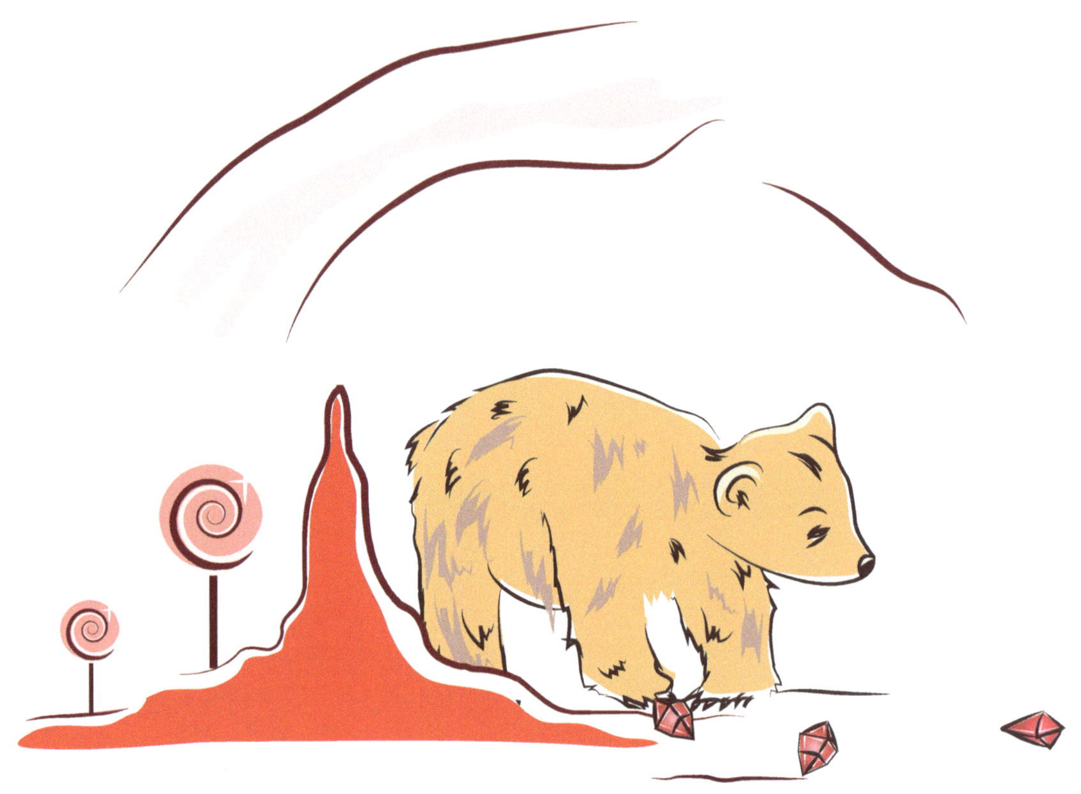

You feel safe and
confident.

Now, Mosey is walking into a new cave.

It is an orange cave. It feels warm.

You see wonderful orange swirls of strength around you.

You warm your hands and **notice all the strength you feel** in this cave.

Mosey is smiling with a warm glow on his face. You **feel stronger and happier** as you walk through the orange cave.

The next cave is yellow.

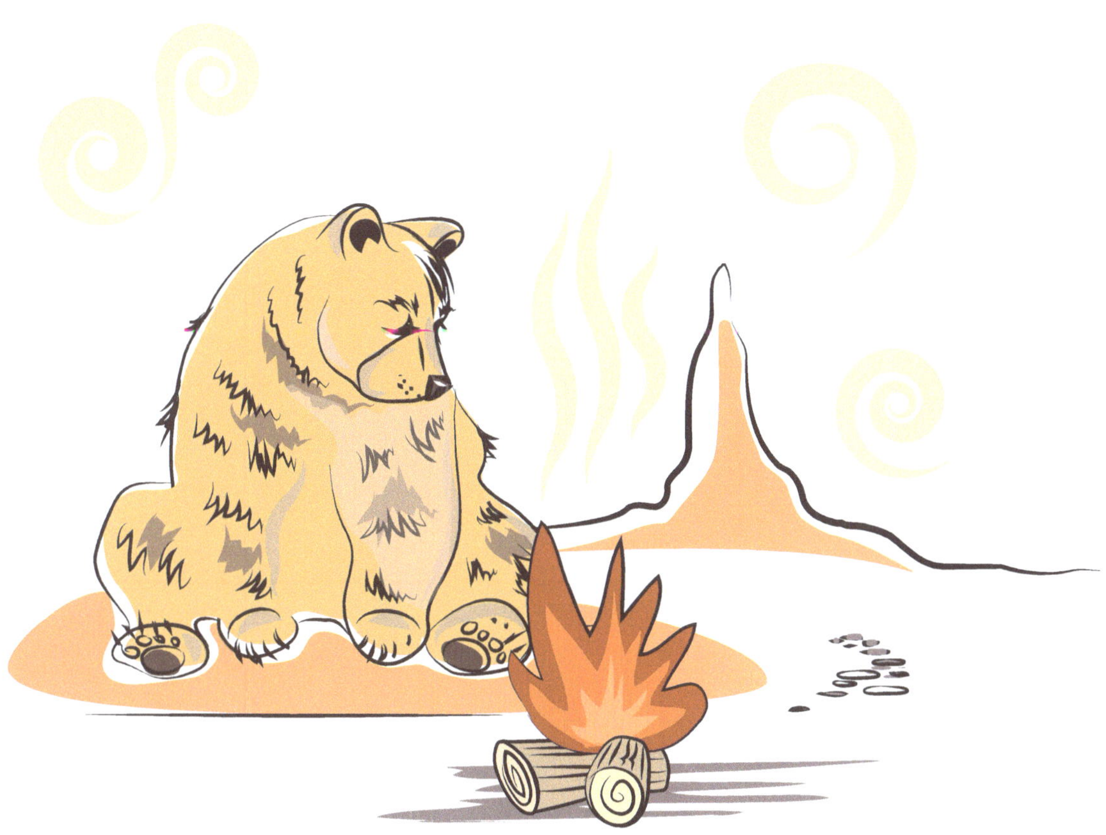

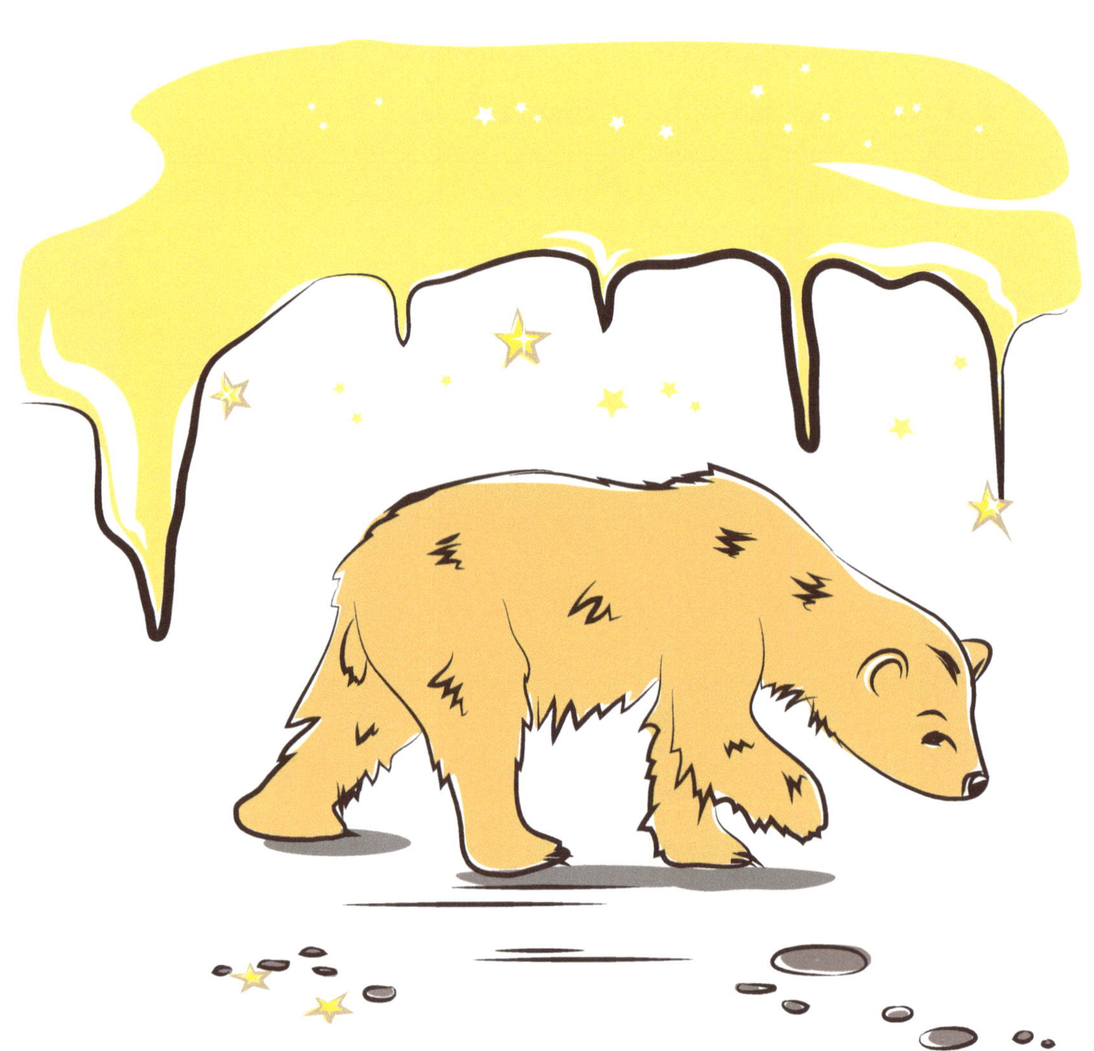

The yellow cave shines brightly just like you! It sparkles like sunshine and fireflies. In here you see special golden stars in the walls. The walls are full are gold stars of wisdom. A special yellow bag appears across your shoulder to put the stars into. Collect some stars. Pick the golden stars you like. Each one has something for you. Ten, nine, eight, seven stars, take as many as you need. Mosey is counting stars. He takes five, four, number three and then you can take what you need.

The bag **feels a bit heavy** with all those stars, and then all the numbers are gone. You have what you need now. So **you know you can move forwards** into the next cave.

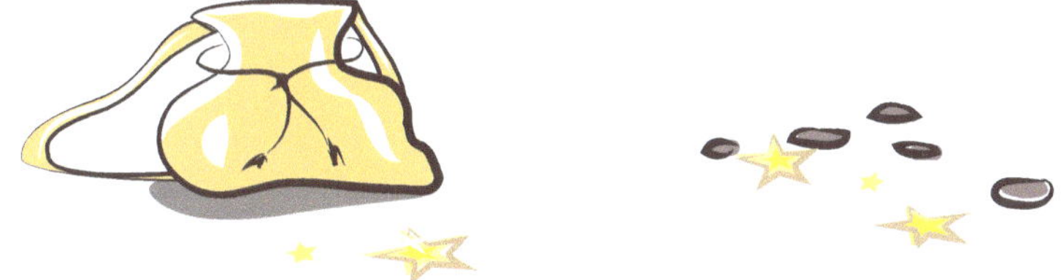

Now up ahead is a green cave.

A sparking rainforest ahead. In here you see lots of green plants, leaves and shoots. You can hear noises of some birds and animals. The green cave is for growth. **You can grow** in here like the green plants, **you can learn** from the plants how they grow when **they have exactly what they need.**

You see a watering can, pick it up and water the plants and they smile back at you. **When you relax you will feel fresh and ready for every moment.** Every plant you see is growing. You breathe in and out, taking deeper breaths as you look around at the beautiful rainforest.

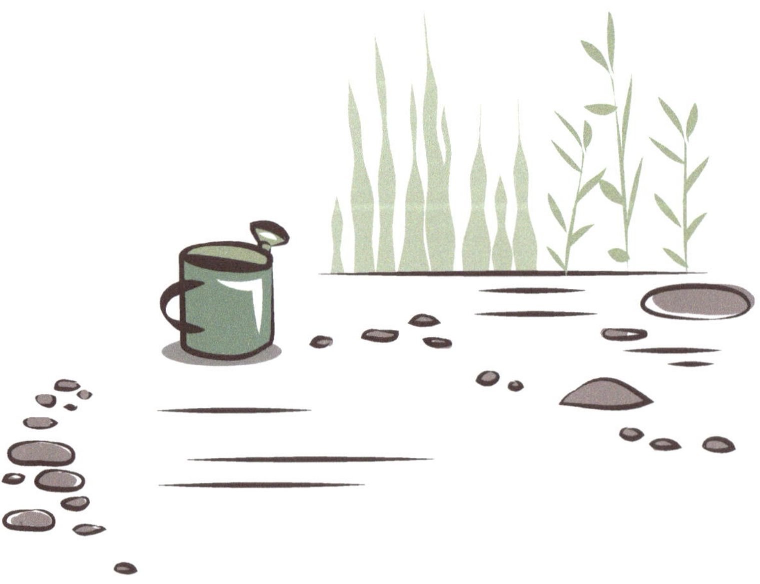

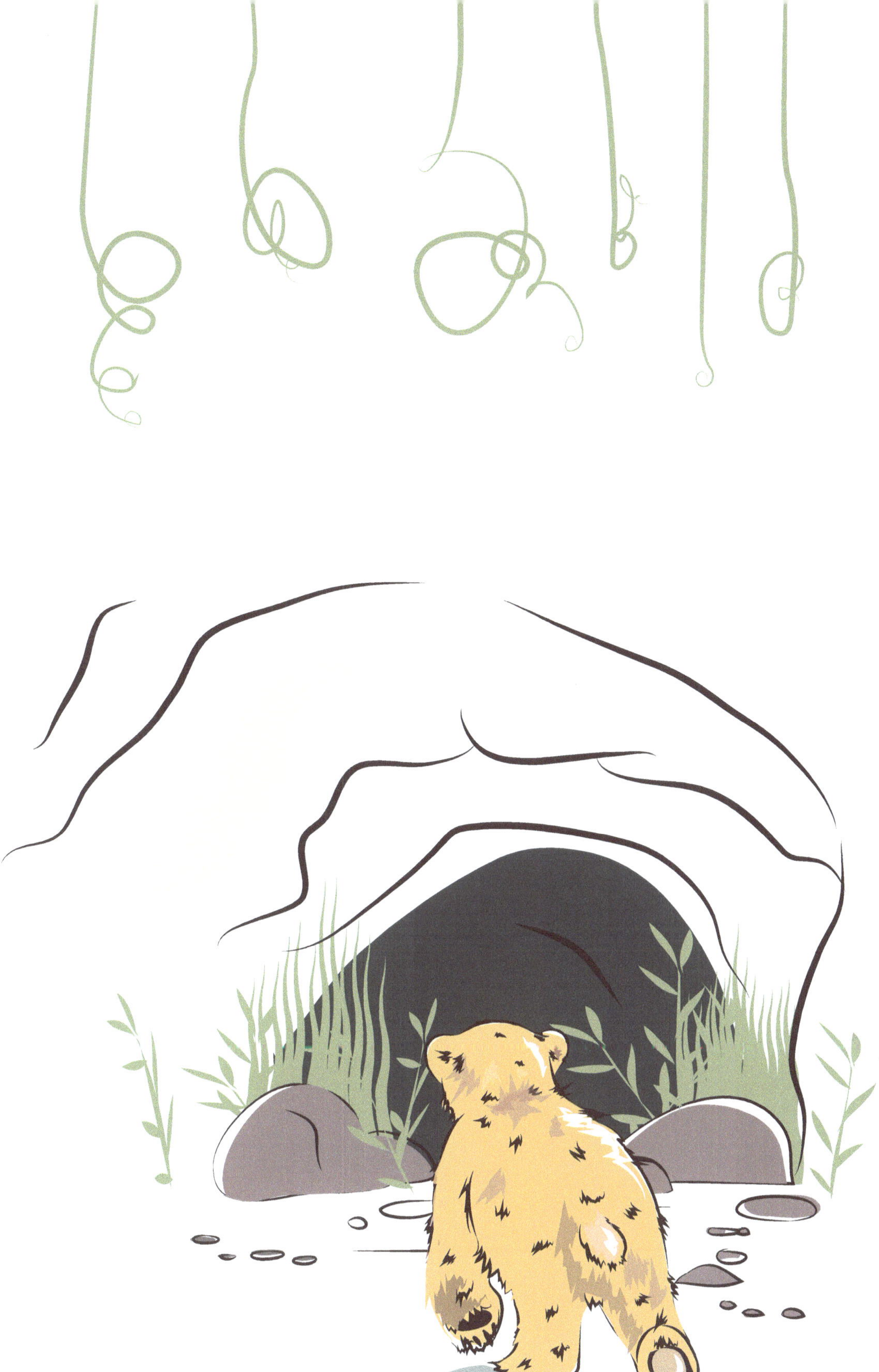

Up ahead is a blue cave. It had a blue glow. You walk in. It has blue pools of water on the ground and water drips down from the walls. It is so calm and peaceful. The water drips; **down, down, down,** calmer and clearer with every drop. **You feel peaceful** here.

It's easy to relax and feel calm and happy. You see Mosey is enjoying the pools too; relaxing in the cool pools of water.

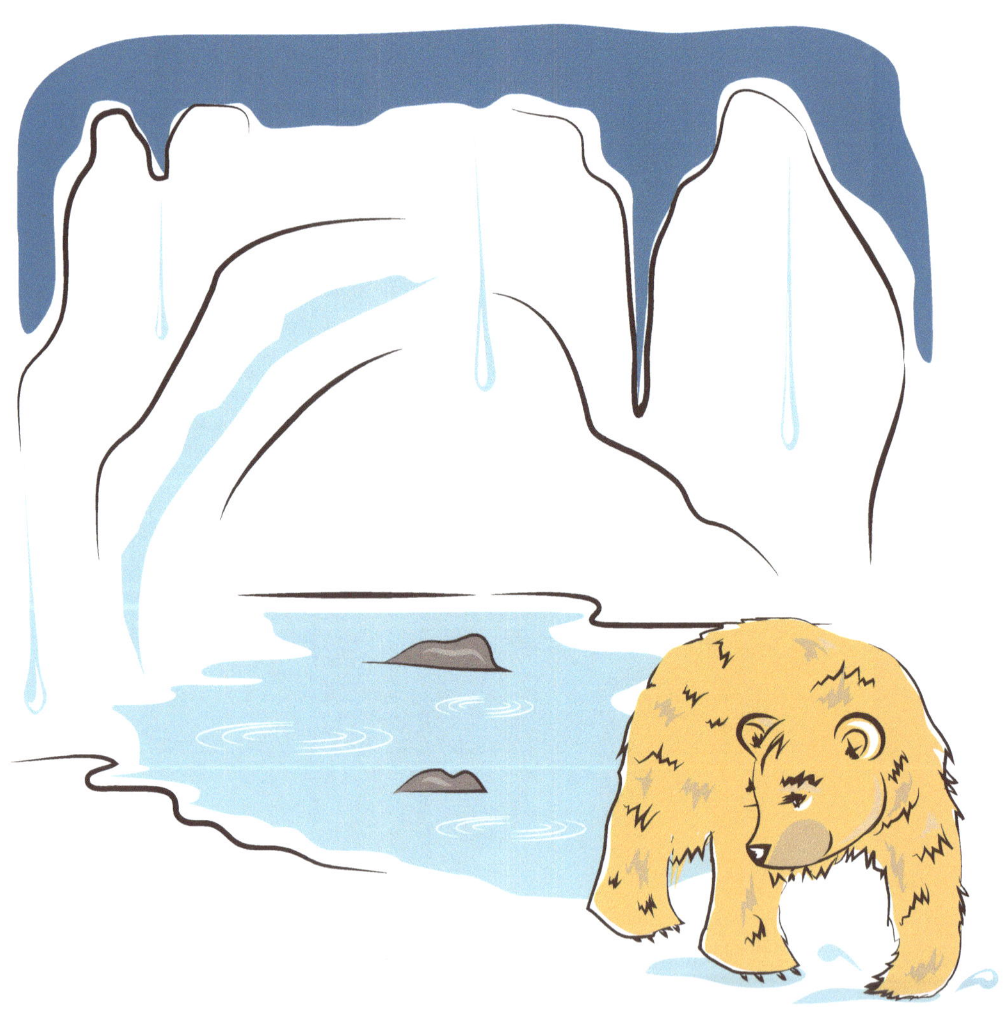

Next is the purple cave of power. You see the purple jewels shining
all over the walls of the purple cave. In here you feel your own special
powers. They can be things you are good at. Special powers can also be
things that you are not good at too. Feel your power in every part of
your body. Take some jewels of wisdom from the walls and put them
in your special bag. The purple cave is pleased that you know you have
the power to do anything you want.
Wander through to the pink cave…

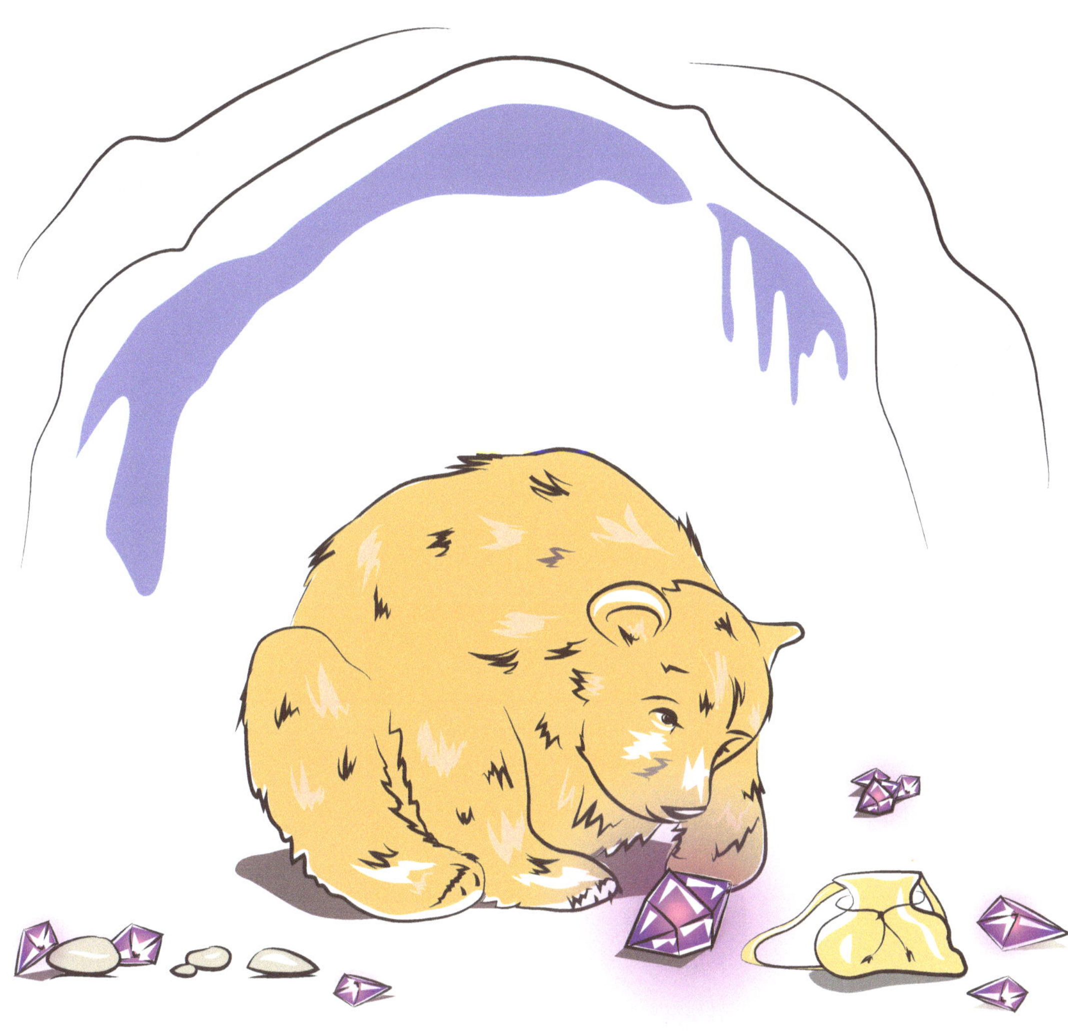

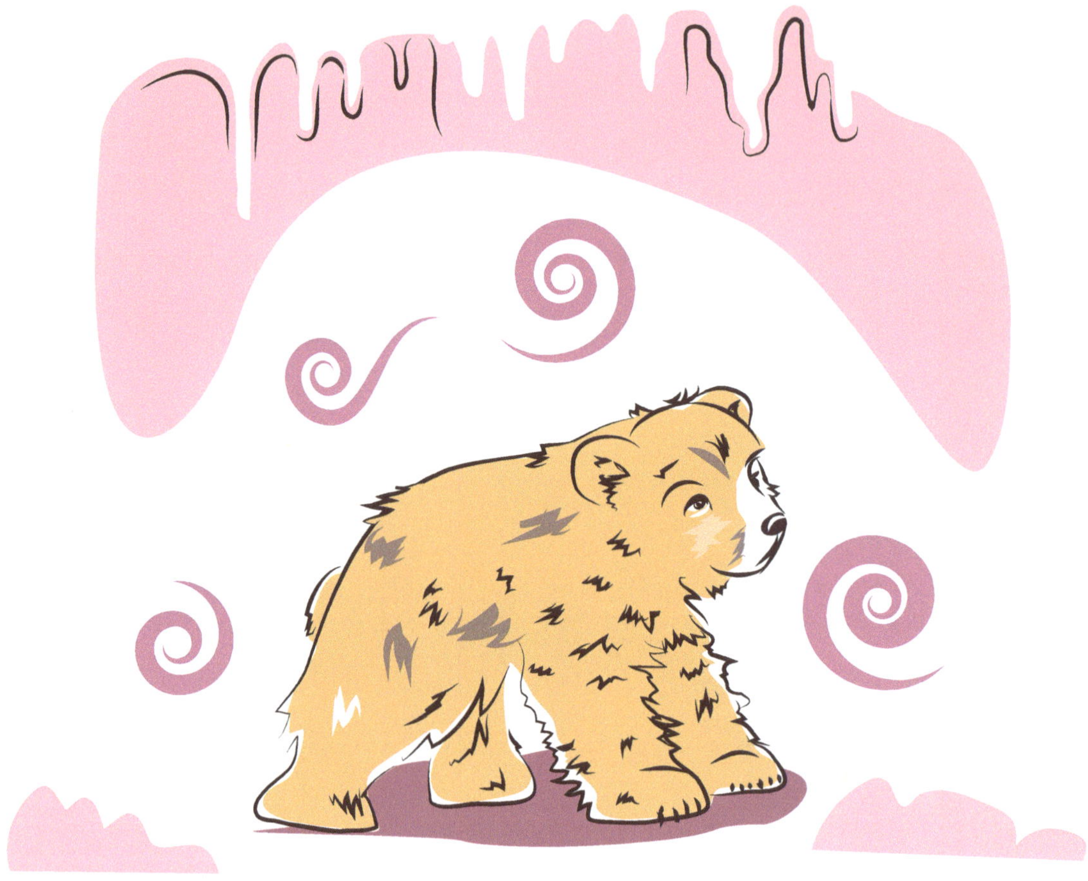

The pink cave is full of kindness and compassion. You can take all the kindness you want in here. Feel it fill your body and mind. The pink cave is fluffy and soft, and brimming with swirls of compassion. It can melt hearts and brings peace and happiness to everyone who visits it. Mosey bear's chest fills with kindness in here. Can you feel your chest filling with kindness too?

Well done Mosey; you have now reached the final cave.
It is the gold Rainbow Cave. It shines a golden glow.

There is a book in the middle of the cave. You go over to it and look at it with Mosey bear. It says, "RELAX" in big letters. Mosey bear opens it and a golden mist blows gently onto his face as he reads. As the mist fills the air, Mosey starts to loosen his body and relax even more. The golden mist fills the special cave and calm golden dust drops gently onto his shoulders.

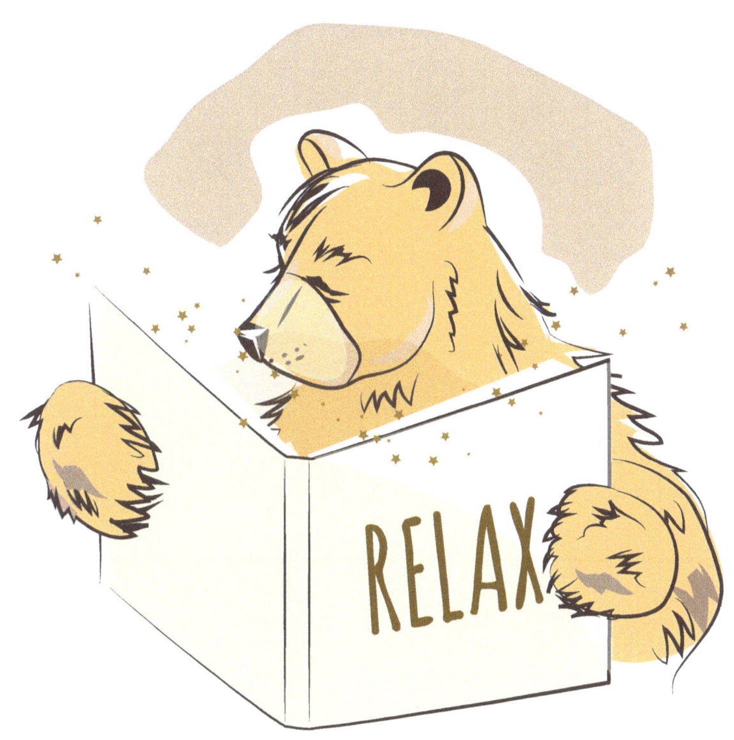

The gold dust is super soft as happiness spreads across his face. You can imagine gold dust spreading across your face too.

You can start your day now, as you feel wonderfully relaxed, with a body and mind ready for anything you are doing today.

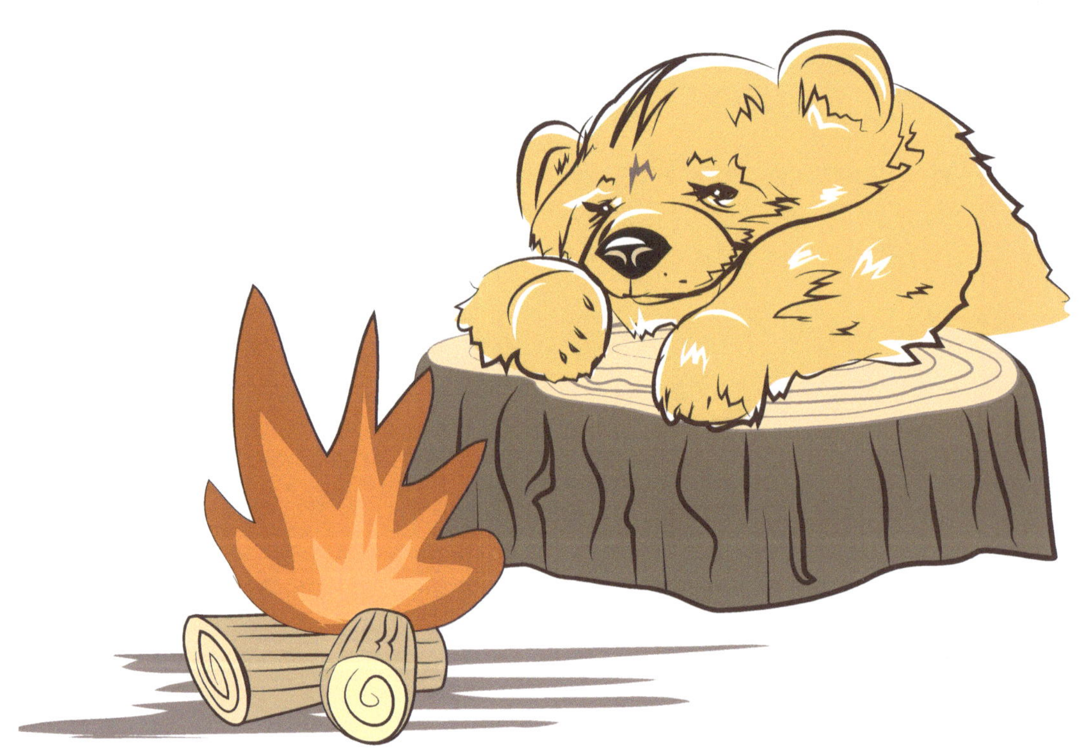

Have a wonderful day; breathe and relax, whatever comes your way!

# Relax and keep calm!

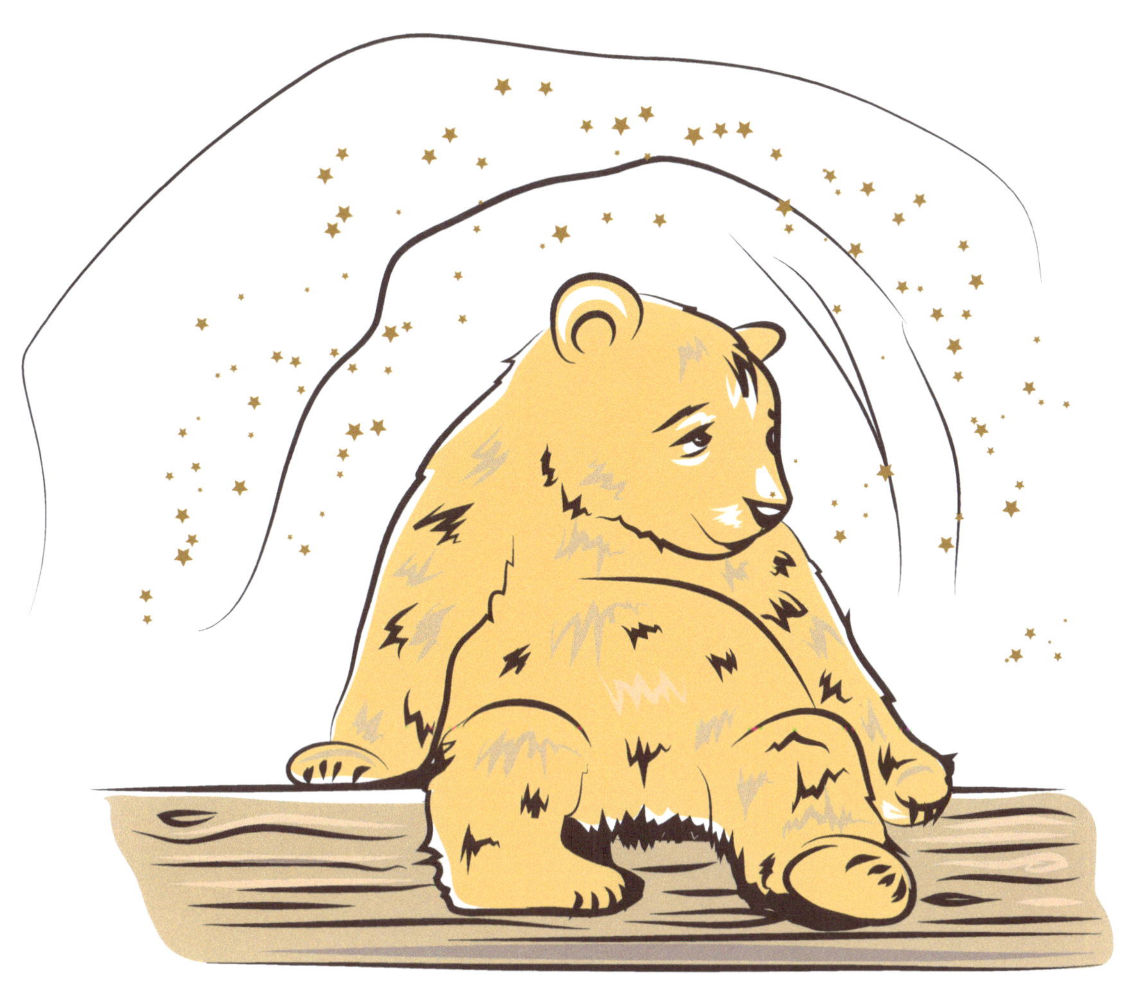

Wow, relaxation is fun and simple!

# Quick relaxation activity!

*We can all relax and feel calm. You can feel calmer wherever you chose.*

Pick a cave now and imagine how calm you feel in your favourite cave. This is the cave you can imagine when you want to relax. You can go there any time you chose.

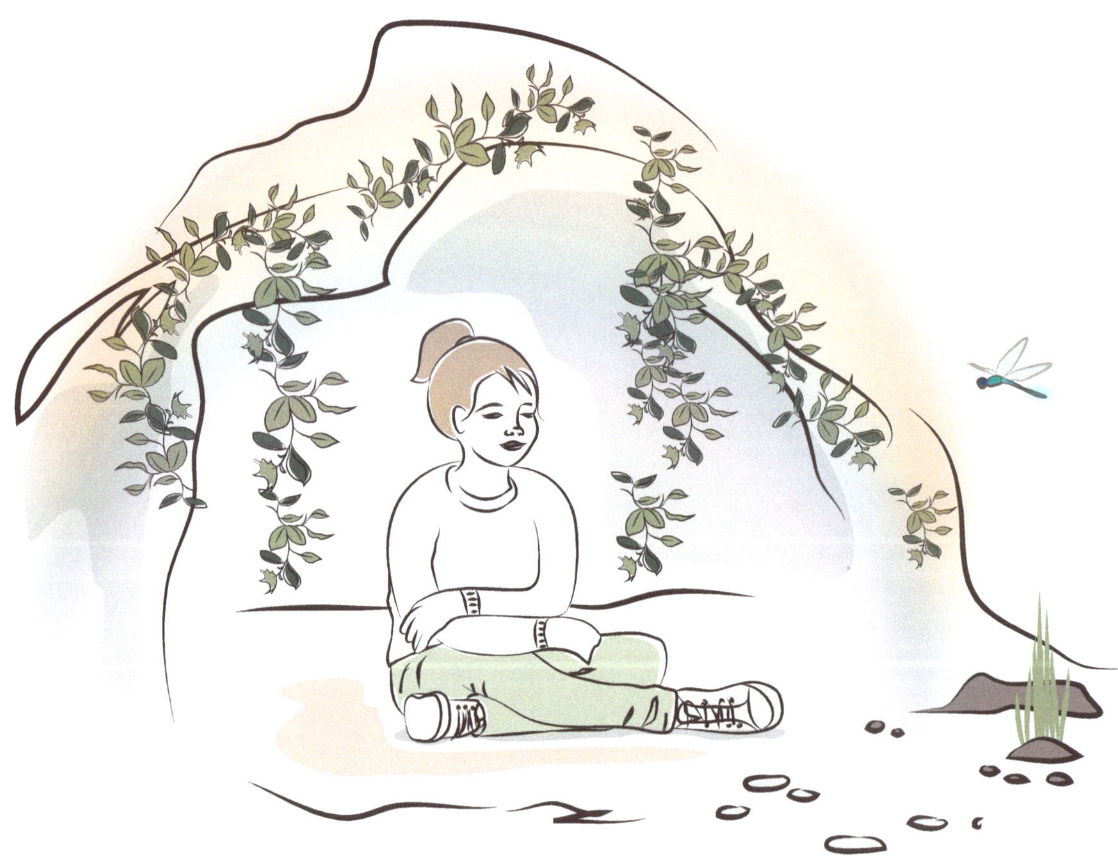

**We will find ourselves able to relax even at difficult moments.**

**We know we can find our special peace over and over again.**

**It's with us when we need it.**

# Things to do

Make a list of places you feel calm and peaceful in.

Think of some imaginary places that make you feel calm.
Eg. A beach, a forest, a boat, a rainbow cave.

Think of words that make you feel calm.
Make a poster of your words.

Think where is the calmest place in your body now?
Check again at different times of the day.
Is there anywhere that feels angry in your body today?
What colour is anger for you?
Can you change the colour to feel calm again?
Can you find your angry spot and make it calm by breathing slowly?
Practice with a friend.

Who makes you feel calm to be with?

What's your favourite relaxing activity?
Walking      Dancing      Reading
Riding a bike      Listening to music
Drawing      Something else?

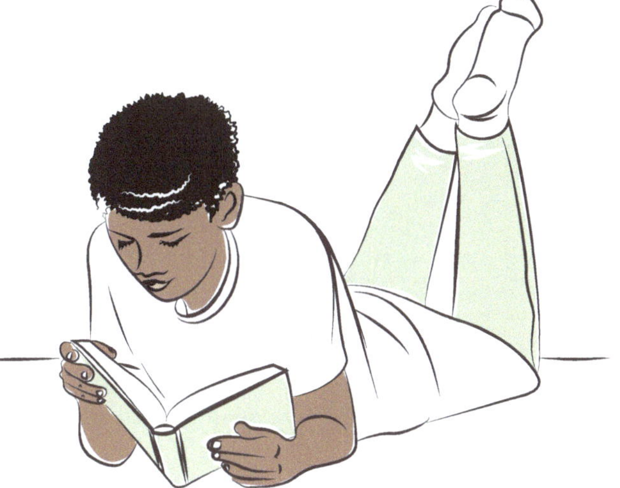

Colour the picture and draw a rainbow above the cave.

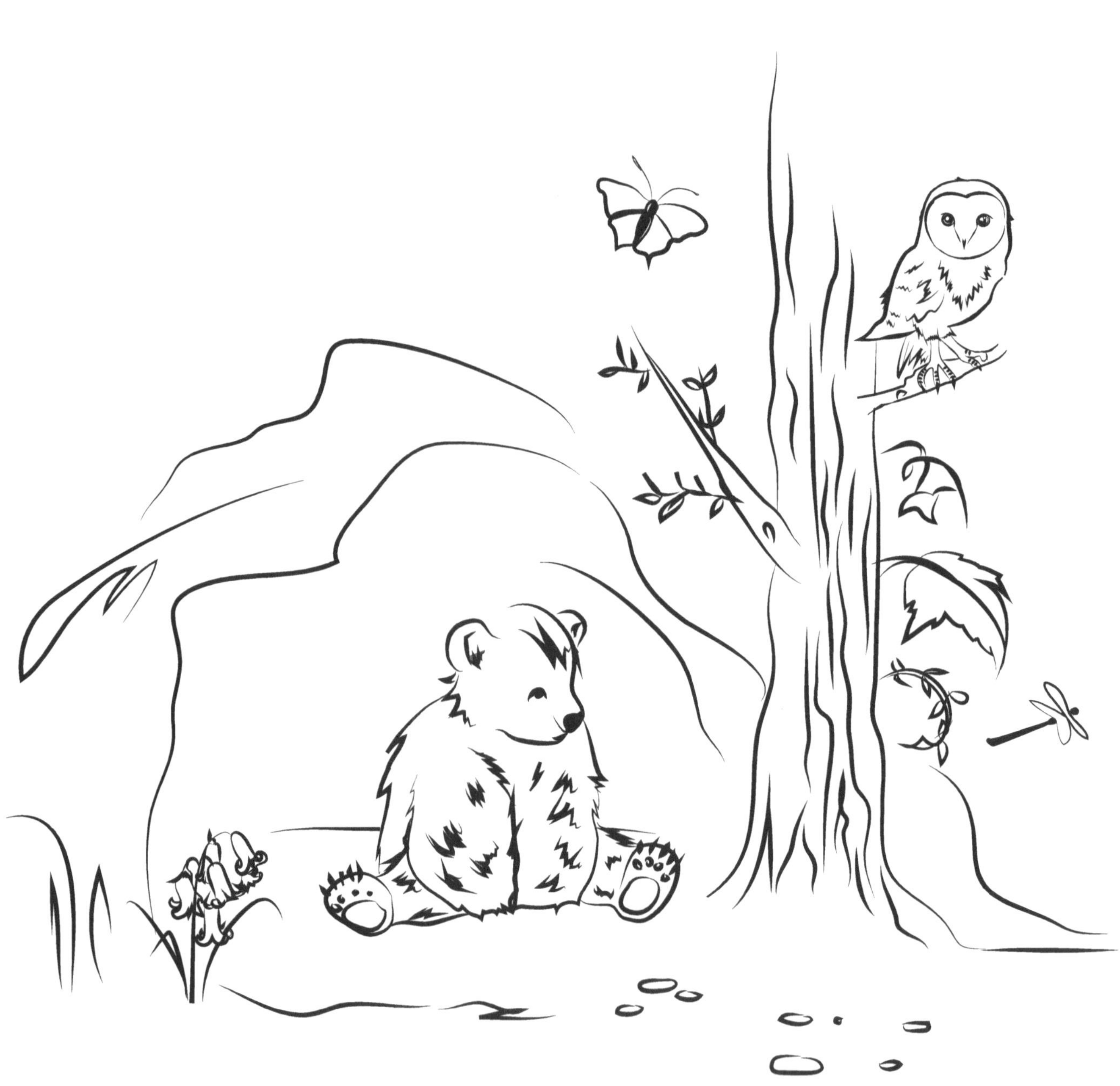

# About the Author

Kate is a teacher, currently working in a complex health class. After gaining a diploma in hypnotherapy and counselling, she has developed psychological approaches in her writing. She is passionate about creativity and behaviour change in health and education.

This book was illustrated by her sister Liz, previously a digital designer now teaching in a SEND school.

*Other books by Kate & Liz Mullin:*
*Pongy Stinkbelly finds a friend*
*A Bear's Sleepy Journey*
*The Lost King*
*Twisted Tales of the Internet*

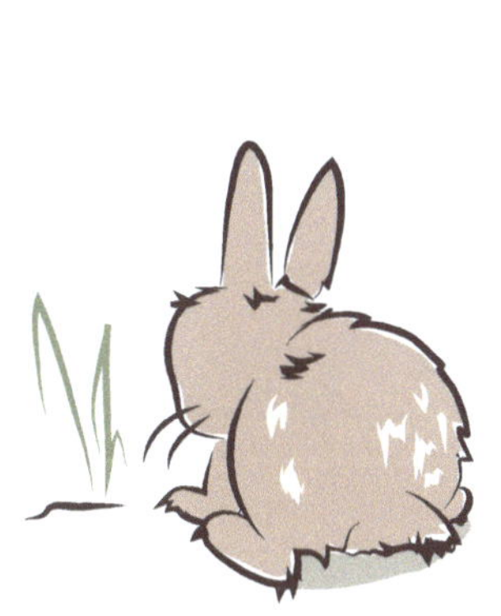

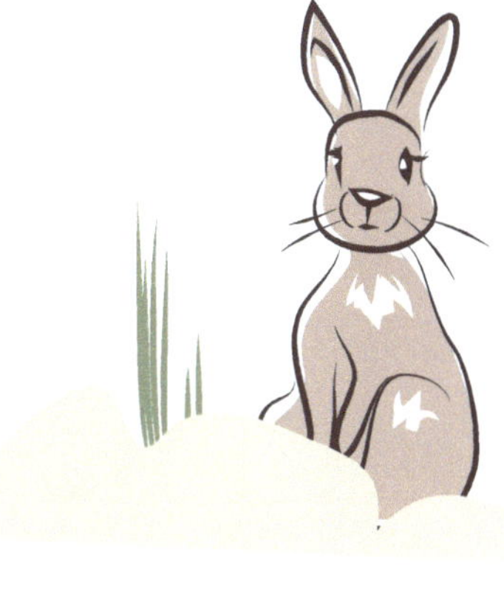

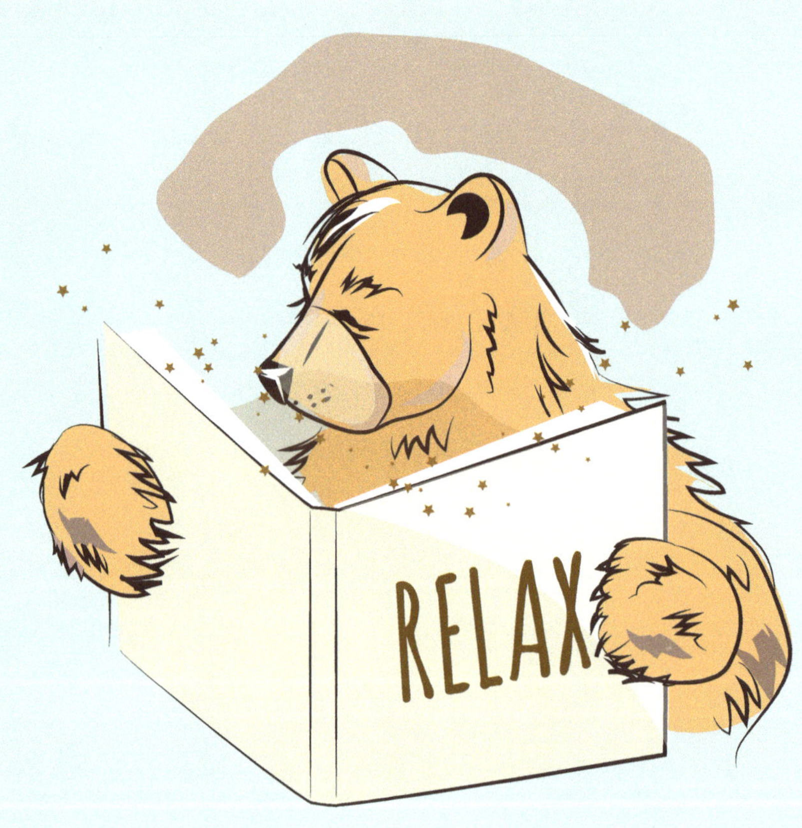


A Relaxation Journey © Copyright 2018